Resistance Band Workouts for Seniors

The Easy-Does-It Strengthener

Helen Talbott

Disclaimer

The information contained in this book is intended for educational purposes only and is not intended to be a substitute for professional medical advice, diagnosis, or treatment. Readers are encouraged to seek the advice of a qualified healthcare professional before starting any new exercise program, especially if they have any pre-existing medical conditions.

The author and publisher of this book disclaim any liability for any injury or damage resulting from the use of the information contained herein.

Important Disclaimer

The Easy-Does-It Strengthener: Resistance Band Workouts for Seniors provides general fitness information and exercise routines designed specifically for older adults. While the information and exercises are presented in a clear and comprehensive manner, it is important to remember that:

- **This book is not a substitute for professional medical advice.** You should always consult with your doctor before starting any new exercise program, especially if you have any pre-existing medical conditions or limitations.
- **Results may vary.** The exercises presented in this book are designed to be safe and effective for most seniors, but individual results may vary depending on age, fitness level, and other factors.
- **Listen to your body.** It is important to pay attention to your body and stop any exercise that causes pain or discomfort.

- **Seek professional guidance if needed.** If you have any concerns or questions, consult with a certified personal trainer, physical therapist, or other qualified healthcare professional.

By using this book, you acknowledge and agree to the following:

- You understand that the information and exercises provided are for informational purposes only and do not constitute medical advice.
- You assume all risks associated with participating in any exercise program.
- You will consult with your doctor before starting any new exercise program.

Enjoy your fitness journey!

Remember, the disclaimer page is crucial to protect yourself and your readers. Adapt this template to your specific content and consult with a legal professional if necessary.

Table of contents

Introduction

Warm-Up & Cool-Down Routines: Preparing Your Body for Success

Mastering Bodyweight Exercises for Form & Control: Building a Strong Foundation

Introduction to Resistance Band Techniques: Unlocking the Power of Bands

Upper Body Power: Arms, Shoulders, & Back - Build Strength and Confidence

Core Strength & Stability: The Powerhouse Within

Lower Body Blast: Legs & Glutes - Sculpt and Strengthen Your Powerhouse

Balance & Coordination Exercises: Mastering Movement with Confidence

Flexibility & Stretching Routines: Unlocking Movement Freedom

Advanced Workout Progressions & Modifications: Pushing Your Limits with Confidence

Staying Motivated & Making Fitness a Habit: Fueling Your Journey to Success

Appendices

Glossary

Bonus

About the author

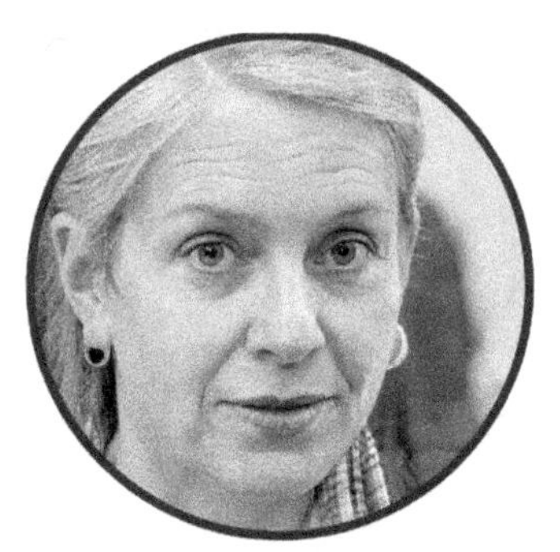

As Helen Talbott, I'm passionate about empowering seniors to embrace an active, fulfilling lifestyle. My journey began after witnessing the limitations firsthand: a dear friend, robbed of her vibrancy by age-related muscle loss, inspired me to explore solutions. I discovered the magic of resistance bands – accessible, adaptable, and incredibly effective for building strength and independence.

Armed with knowledge and enthusiasm, I embarked on a mission to share this empowering tool with others. I devoured research, collaborated with fitness experts, and carefully crafted resistance band routines tailored specifically for seniors. My philosophy is simple: **easy-does-it, yet impactful**. Small, consistent steps lead to remarkable results, boosting strength, improving balance, and rekindling the joy of movement.

Through Helen Talbott, I guide you on this journey – not as a distant expert, but as a supportive friend. This book is your personalized road map, filled with clear instructions, modifications, and encouraging wisdom. It's more than just exercises; it's a celebration of your potential, a reminder that staying active at any age is not only possible, but truly empowering.

Beyond the book:

- I regularly speak at senior centers and workshops, sharing my knowledge and motivating others to embrace an active lifestyle.
- I'm constantly exploring new ways to make fitness accessible and enjoyable for every senior, always seeking the latest research and techniques.

Join me on this journey – let's unlock the strength and confidence within, together!

Introduction

Forget the dumbbells and treadmills – it's time to embrace the Easy-Does-It Strengthener: your ultimate guide to getting fit and vibrant with resistance bands! No matter your age, activity level, or past experiences, this book is your invitation to unleash your inner champion and discover the joy of building strength in a safe, effective, and downright fun way.

Ditch the doubts, forget the limitations. Whether you're yearning for more energy to keep up with the grandkids, dreaming of tackling that garden with ease, or simply want to feel stronger and more confident, this book is your passport to a healthier, happier you. **No need for**

intimidating gyms or complicated routines. We'll equip you with the knowledge and exercises to transform your fitness journey from daunting to delightful.

Think colorful bands, not bulky weights. We'll introduce you to the magic of resistance bands, your new best friends that fit practically anywhere, adapt to any fitness level, and offer a gentle yet powerful challenge. **Think pain-free progress, not pushing yourself to the limit.** We'll focus on safe, effective exercises that respect your body's unique needs and limitations, all while delivering results you can see and feel.

This isn't just about exercise, it's about empowerment. We'll guide you through every step, from choosing the right bands to mastering proper form, crafting personalized workout plans, and staying motivated along the way. **Get ready to unlock a newfound sense of strength, confidence, and independence.** With each band loop, you'll be building not just muscles, but a brighter, more vibrant future.

So, are you ready to **embrace the Easy-Does-It Strengthener** and embark on a journey of strength, vitality, and joy? Turn the page and let's begin!

Why Resistance Bands Are the Perfect Match for Active Seniors:

Forget hefty weights and intimidating gyms, seniors seeking to build strength and improve fitness can rejoice! Resistance bands offer a safe, effective, and surprisingly fun way to stay active and reap a multitude of benefits, making them the perfect match for the older adult fitness enthusiast. Here's why:

Gentle on the Joints:

- Unlike free weights or machines, resistance bands provide constant, even tension throughout the movement, minimizing stress on joints prone to wear and tear. This allows for pain-free exercise and a lower risk of injury.

Adjustable Intensity:

- Forget feeling overwhelmed! The beauty of resistance bands lies in their versatility. By simply choosing different bands or varying loops and grips, you can easily adjust the intensity of your workout, tailoring it to your individual fitness level and needs.

Convenient & Portable:

- Who needs a gym membership? Resistance bands are compact, lightweight, and travel-friendly. You can easily stash them in your purse, suitcase, or even under the couch, allowing you to work out anywhere, anytime.

Functional Strength:

- Unlike machines that isolate specific muscles, resistance bands mimic everyday movements, engaging multiple muscle groups and promoting functional strength. This translates to improved balance, coordination, and daily activities like carrying groceries or climbing stairs.

Variety & Fun:

- Forget stale routines! Resistance bands offer a vast array of exercises targeting all major muscle groups, from bicep curls and squats to chest presses and rows. You can easily mix and match, keeping your workouts fresh and engaging.

Safety & Control:

- The controlled tension of resistance bands allows for proper form and technique, minimizing the risk of improper alignment and injury. This is especially important for seniors who may be new to exercise or have specific needs.

Improved Bone Density & Reduced Osteoporosis:

- Studies show that resistance training with bands can increase bone mineral density, decreasing the risk of osteoporosis, a common concern for older adults.

Overall Health & Well-being:

- Regular exercise with resistance bands has numerous benefits for seniors, including improved cardiovascular health, weight management, better sleep, and even cognitive function.

With their ease of use, adaptability, and plethora of benefits, resistance bands offer a unique and empowering way for seniors to stay active, build strength, and improve their overall well-being. So, grab your bands and get ready to experience the "Easy-Does-It Strengthener" advantage!

Getting Started: Choosing the Right Bands and Setting Up Your Environment

Welcome to the exciting world of resistance band workouts! Before you dive into sculpting your strength, let's navigate the essentials of getting started.

Choosing Your Band Buddies:

- **Resistance Levels:** Don't be intimidated! Bands come in a variety of resistances, typically labeled by color or weight equivalent. Start light and gradually progress. Lighter bands (yellow, green) are great for beginners or specific exercises, while heavier bands (red, blue) offer more challenge.
- **Material:** Latex or fabric? Latex bands offer more resistance, while fabric bands are gentler on skin and easier to grip. Choose what feels best for you.
- **Type of Band:** Consider your goals. Loop bands are versatile for various exercises. Door anchor bands offer more stability for

seated exercises. Mini bands target specific muscle groups.

Creating Your Fitness Oasis:

- **Find Your Space:** Pick a well-lit, clutter-free area with enough space to move freely without bumping into furniture. Ensure good ventilation, especially for more vigorous workouts.
- **Comfort is Key:** Invest in a supportive exercise mat to cushion your joints and provide traction. Wear comfortable clothing that allows for unrestricted movement.
- **Hydration Station:** Keep a water bottle handy to stay hydrated throughout your workout.
- **Safety First:** Ensure you have good footing by using a non-slip mat or workout shoes. Inform your doctor before starting any new exercise program, especially if you have any health concerns.

Tips for Band Selection:

- **Start conservative:** Choose lighter bands initially and progress gradually to avoid strain.
- **Test the tension:** Before starting your workout, test each band by pulling it gently to gauge its resistance and ensure it's comfortable.
- **Consider your goals:** If targeting specific muscle groups, consider mini bands. Door anchor bands offer stability for seated exercises.
- **Consult a professional:** If unsure, seek guidance from a certified trainer or physical therapist to help you choose the right bands and exercises.

Remember: Setting up your environment promotes focus and enjoyment. With the right bands and a comfortable space, you're ready to embark on your resistance band adventure!

Important Safety Tips for Senior Exercisers:

Embracing an active lifestyle with resistance bands is fantastic! However, prioritizing safety remains paramount, especially for older adults. Here are some key tips to keep you moving with confidence:

Listen to Your Body:

- **Start slow and progress gradually:** Avoid overexertion. Begin with shorter workouts and lighter bands, increasing intensity and duration as you gain strength.
- **Pay attention to pain:** It's a signal to stop! Modify exercises or rest if you experience any discomfort. Pain should never be part of a workout.
- **Warm-up and cool-down:** Prepare your muscles with gentle stretches and light movement before your workout, and wind down with cool-down stretches.
- **Stay hydrated:** Drink plenty of water before, during, and after your workout to

prevent dehydration, especially in hot environments.

Prioritize Proper Form:

- **Focus on technique:** Use proper form for each exercise to ensure you activate the right muscles and avoid injury. If unsure, consult a certified trainer or physical therapist.
- **Maintain good posture:** Keep your back straight, core engaged, and shoulders relaxed throughout your exercises.
- **Control your movements:** Avoid jerky motions and focus on smooth, controlled movements.
- **Don't hold your breath:** Breathe steadily and rhythmically throughout your exercises.

Embrace Safety Practices:

- **Clear your workout area:** Ensure your space is free of clutter and tripping hazards.

- **Wear supportive shoes:** Invest in proper footwear with good traction to prevent falls.
- **Use a non-slip mat:** Especially important for floor exercises to minimize the risk of slipping.
- **Work out with a partner or inform someone:** This provides safety support and peace of mind, especially if you live alone.
- **Monitor your health:** Consult your doctor before starting any new exercise program, especially if you have any health conditions.

Additional Tips:

- **Listen to your limitations:** Know your current fitness level and don't push yourself beyond your capabilities.
- **Modify exercises:** Adapt exercises to your abilities and limitations. There are always modifications available!

- **Take breaks:** Don't be afraid to rest when needed. Listen to your body and take breaks as needed.
- **Celebrate your progress:** Focus on your achievements, no matter how small, and be proud of your commitment to staying active.

Remember, the goal is to enjoy exercise and improve your well-being safely. By following these tips and listening to your body, you can reap the numerous benefits of resistance band workouts while minimizing the risk of injury. So, let's get moving confidently!

Benefits of Resistance band

Resistance bands offer numerous benefits for everyone, but especially for seniors looking to stay active and healthy. Here are some key advantages:

Gentle on Joints: Unlike free weights or machines, resistance bands provide constant, even tension throughout the movement, minimizing stress on joints prone to wear and tear. This allows for pain-free exercise and a lower risk of injury.

Adjustable Intensity: No matter your fitness level, you can find the perfect challenge. Simply choose different bands or vary loops and grips to adapt the intensity to your needs.

Convenient & Portable: Take your workout anywhere! Bands are compact, lightweight, and travel-friendly, allowing you to exercise at home, the park, or even on vacation.

Functional Strength: Unlike machines that isolate specific muscles, resistance bands mimic everyday movements, engaging multiple muscle groups and promoting functional strength. This means improved balance, coordination, and daily activities like carrying groceries or climbing stairs.

Variety & Fun: Ditch the stale routines! Bands offer a vast array of exercises targeting all major muscle groups, keeping your workouts fresh and engaging.

Safety & Control: The controlled tension allows for proper form and technique, minimizing the risk of improper alignment and injury. This is especially important for seniors who may be new to exercise or have specific needs.

Improved Bone Density & Reduced Osteoporosis: Studies show that resistance training with bands can increase bone mineral density, decreasing the risk of osteoporosis, a common concern for older adults.

Overall Health & Well-being: Regular exercise with resistance bands has numerous benefits for seniors, including improved cardiovascular health, weight management, better sleep, and even cognitive function.

Part 1

Building the Basics

Chapter 1

Warm-Up & Cool-Down Routines: Preparing Your Body for Success

Imagine your body as a symphony orchestra. Before a grand performance, the instruments need to tune up – warming up your muscles before exercise is just as crucial. Just like a proper cool-down ensures the instruments wind down gently, it helps your body gradually return to its resting state. This chapter equips you with effective warm-up and cool-down routines specifically designed for active seniors using resistance bands.

Why Warm Up?

Preparing your muscles with a proper warm-up offers several benefits:

- **Increased blood flow:** Warms up your muscles, improves oxygen delivery, and prepares them for activity.
- **Improved flexibility:** Loosens your joints and increases range of motion, minimizing risk of injury.
- **Enhanced mental focus:** Gets you mentally prepared for your workout and improves coordination.
- **Reduced risk of injury:** Minimizes muscle strains and tears by gently preparing them for exercise.

The Perfect Warm-Up:

Here's a simple, effective warm-up routine for seniors using resistance bands:

5-10 minutes of light cardio: Choose activities you enjoy, like brisk walking, jogging in place, or marching with arm swings.

Dynamic stretches: Unlike static stretches, these involve gentle movements, incorporating movement patterns used in your workout. Examples include:

- **Arm circles:** Forward and backward arm circles, gradually increasing size and speed.
- **Leg swings:** Swing each leg forward and backward, keeping your core engaged.
- **Band walks:** Loop a band around your ankles and walk forward and backward, activating leg muscles.

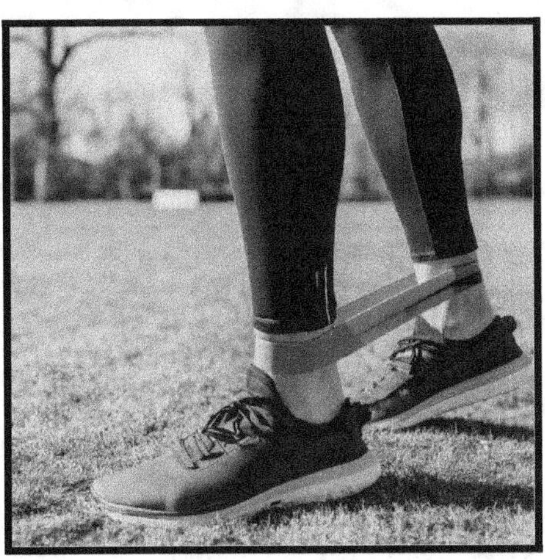

- **Arm swings with bands:** Hold light bands and perform side-to-side arm swings.

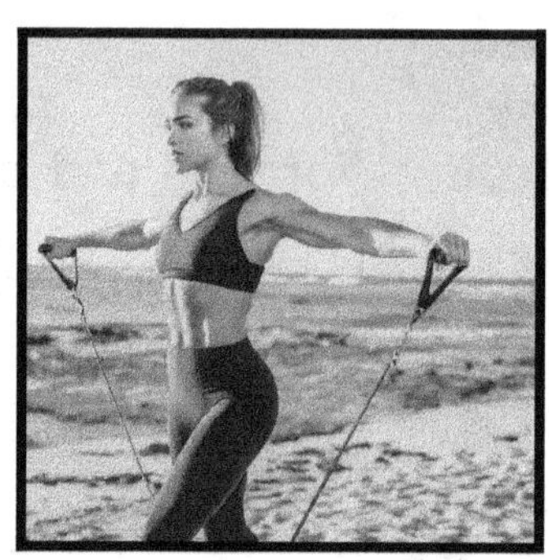

Band-specific warm-up: Perform light exercises using your chosen resistance bands, mimicking movements used in your workout without adding significant weight.

Remember: Listen to your body. Start slowly, gradually increase intensity, and don't push yourself to the point of pain.

Cool-Down: Calming the Symphony

Just like winding down after a performance, a proper cool-down is essential:

- **5-10 minutes of light cardio:** Continue with low-intensity activities like walking, gradually slowing down until you come to a stop.
- **Static stretches:** Hold gentle stretches for 15-30 seconds each, focusing on the major muscle groups used in your workout. Examples include:
- **Hamstring stretch:** Sit on the floor, legs extended, reach towards your toes with a band around your feet.

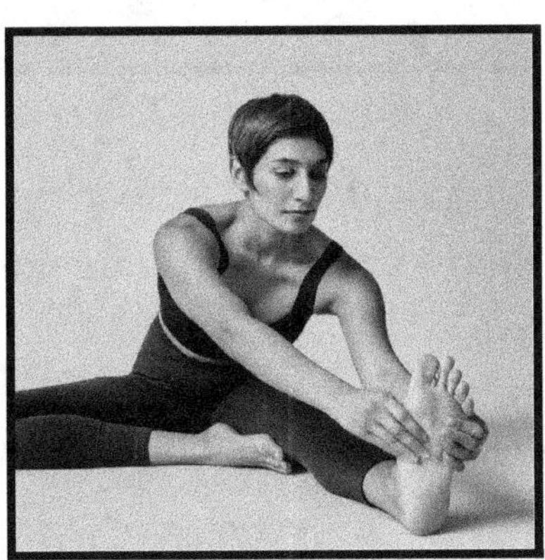

- **Quad stretch:** Stand on one leg, hold a band behind your ankle, and gently pull your heel towards your gluteus.

- **Chest stretch:** Hold a band in front of you, palms facing each other, and gently pull your arms apart.

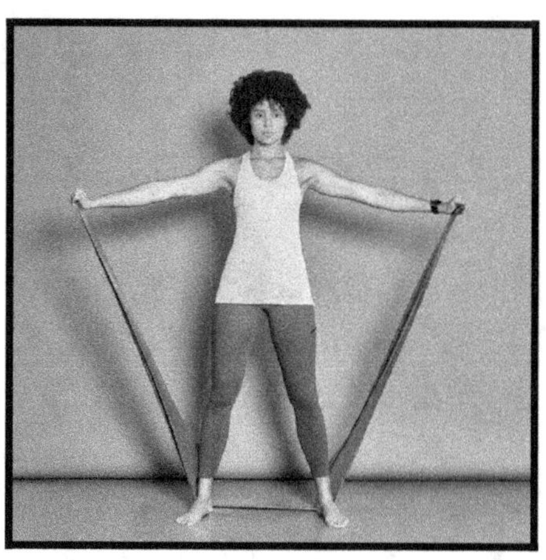

Deep breathing: Take slow, deep breaths for 2-3 minutes to help your heart rate and breathing return to normal.

Tips for Success:

- Warm up in a warm environment to further improve muscle flexibility.
- Stay hydrated throughout your warm-up, workout, and cool-down.

- Modify exercises based on your individual needs and limitations.
- Don't skip the cool-down – it's just as important as the warm-up!

By incorporating these warm-up and cool-down routines into your resistance band workouts, you'll prepare your body for success, minimize the risk of injury, and maximize your enjoyment of exercise. Remember, consistency is key – make these routines a regular part of your fitness journey to feel your best and achieve your goals!

Chapter 2

Mastering Bodyweight Exercises for Form & Control: Building a Strong Foundation

Welcome to the foundation of your fitness journey! Before diving into the world of resistance bands, mastering bodyweight exercises is crucial for building a strong foundation and ensuring proper form and control when adding bands. Think of it as building a sturdy house – before adding fancy features, a solid base is essential for stability and safety.

Why Bodyweight Exercises?

Bodyweight exercises offer numerous benefits:

- **Accessible:** No equipment needed, making them perfect for home workouts or travel.

- **Functional:** Target major muscle groups and mimic everyday movements, improving daily activities.
- **Scalable:** Modify exercises to your fitness level, making them suitable for beginners and experienced exercisers alike.
- **Focus on Form:** Emphasize proper technique without adding external weight, minimizing risk of injury.

Mastering the Basics:

This chapter focuses on key bodyweight exercises for seniors, emphasizing proper form and control:

Squats:

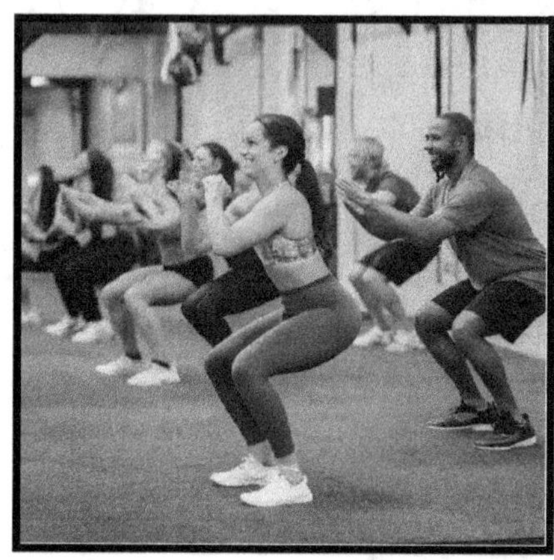

- Stand with feet hip-width apart, toes slightly outward.
- Engage your core and slowly lower your body as if sitting back in a chair.
- Keep your back straight, knees over toes, and heels flat on the ground.
- Stand back up, squeezing your glutes at the top.
- **Modification:** Use a chair for support or perform wall squats, leaning against a wall.

Lunges:

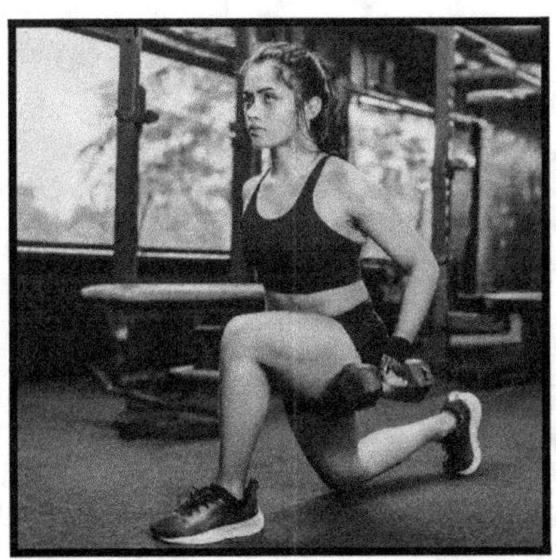

- Stand with feet hip-width apart.
- Step forward with one leg, lowering your body until both knees are bent at 90-degree angles.
- Keep your back straight, front knee over ankle, and rear heel lifted.
- Push back up to starting position, engaging your front leg muscles.
- Repeat on the other side.
- **Modification:** Use a chair for support or perform walking lunges.

Push-ups:

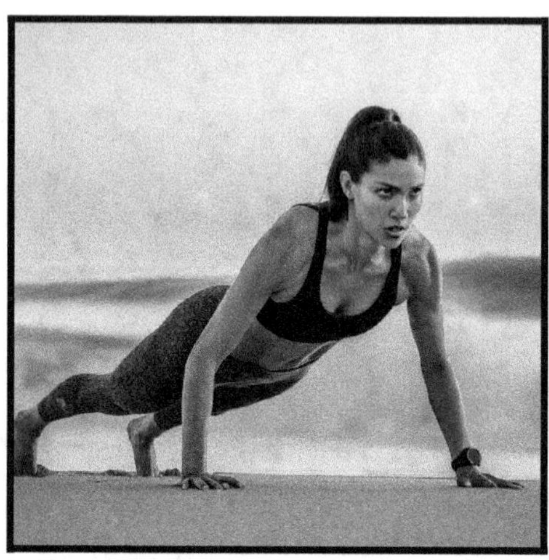

- Start in a plank position with hands shoulder-width apart, body forming a straight line from head to heels.
- Lower your chest towards the ground, bending your elbows and keeping your core engaged.
- Maintain a straight back and avoid letting your hips sag.
- Push back up to starting position.
- **Modification:** Perform modified push-ups on your knees, against a wall, or elevated on a stable surface.

Rows:

- Stand with feet hip-width apart, knees slightly bent, and hold a heavy book or water bottle in each hand.
- Hinge at your hips, leaning forward while keeping your back straight.
- Pull your elbows back towards your sides, squeezing your shoulder blades together.
- Lower the weights back down slowly.
- **Modification:** Use lighter weights or perform seated rows using a chair for support.

Plank

- Start in a push-up position with forearms on the ground.
- Engage your core to keep your body in a straight line from head to heels.
- Hold for as long as you can comfortably without compromising form.
- **Modification:** Perform a plank on your knees or a modified plank against a wall.

Remember:

- Focus on proper form over speed or repetitions.
- Listen to your body and take breaks when needed.
- Breathe steadily throughout each exercise.
- Modify exercises as needed to suit your fitness level and limitations.

Benefits of Mastering Bodyweight Exercises:

- Develop balance, coordination, and core strength.
- Build foundational strength for more advanced resistance band exercises.
- Improve posture and stability.
- Increase bone density and reduce osteoporosis risk.
- Provide a safe and effective workout option.

Moving Forward:

This chapter equips you with the essential bodyweight exercises to build a strong foundation. Remember, consistency is key. Practice these exercises regularly to master your form and control before adding resistance bands in the next chapter. With dedication and this solid foundation, you'll be ready to conquer your fitness goals!

Embrace the journey, master the basics, and get ready to unlock your full potential with resistance bands!

Chapter 3

Introduction to Resistance Band Techniques: Unlocking the Power of Bands

Now that you've mastered bodyweight exercises and understand the importance of proper form, let's unlock the exciting world of resistance band techniques! This chapter will equip you with the knowledge and skills to utilize your bands effectively, maximizing your workouts and achieving your fitness goals.

Understanding Band Mechanics:

- **Tension is key:** Unlike weights, bands offer variable resistance throughout the movement, increasing as you stretch them further. This constant tension engages muscles throughout the entire exercise.
- **Grips and Loops:** Experiment with different grips and loop positions to target

specific muscle groups and vary the intensity of your exercises.

- **Activation & Control:** Focus on controlled movements, feeling the muscles you're engaging, and maintaining proper form over speed or repetitions.

Essential Techniques:

- **Anchoring:** Learn how to securely anchor your bands to doors, poles, or even your own body to add variety and stability to your workouts.
- **Isolations & Combinations:** Discover exercises targeting specific muscle groups (isolations) and compound exercises engaging multiple groups simultaneously.
- **Progressions & Modifications:** Learn how to gradually increase the difficulty of exercises by using different bands, loops, or varying your technique. Adapt exercises to suit your fitness level and limitations.

- **Safety First:** Maintain proper form, listen to your body, and don't hesitate to modify exercises as needed.

Sample Techniques:

- **Bicep Curls:** Anchor the band under your feet, hold the ends, and perform bicep curls, feeling the tension in your arms.

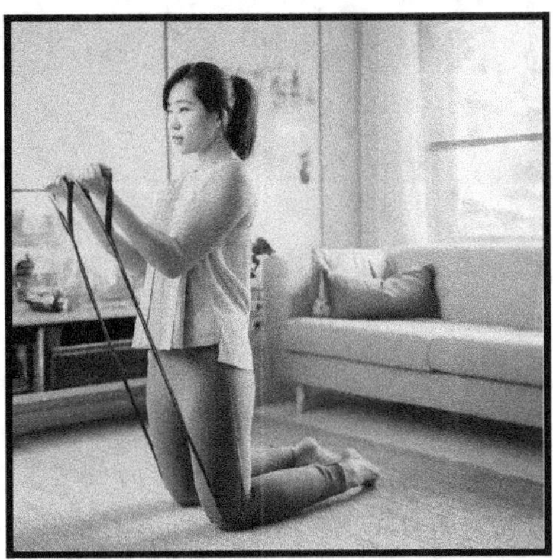

- **Rows:** Sit or stand with the band anchored behind you, pull towards your chest, engaging your back muscles.

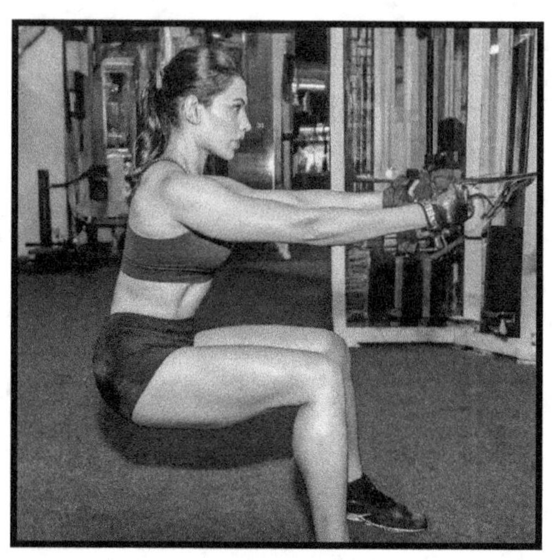

- **Squats with Band:** Loop the band around your thighs just above your knees, perform squats, feeling the added resistance.

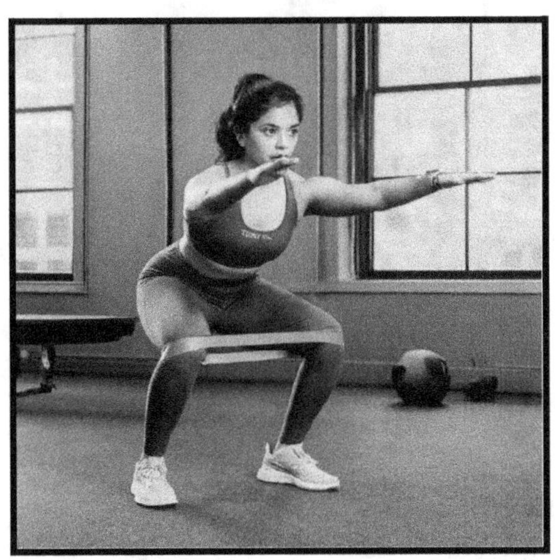

- **Overhead Press:** Loop the band overhead, press your arms up, focusing on your shoulders and triceps.

- **Side Shuffles:** Loop the band around your ankles, perform side shuffles, targeting your hips and glutes.

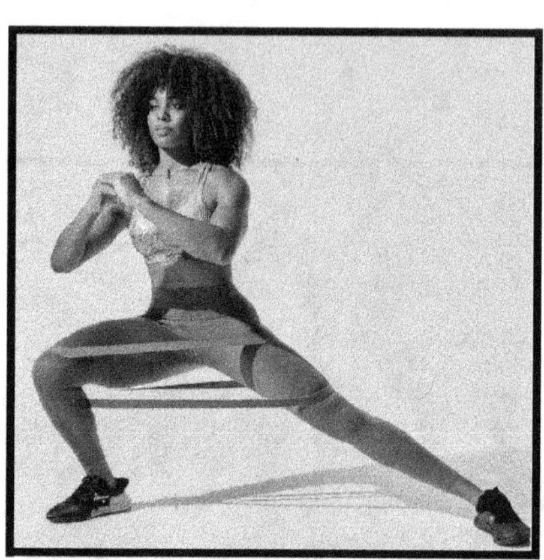

Benefits of Mastering Techniques:

- Increase workout variety and prevent plateaus.
- Target specific muscle groups for balanced development.
- Gradually progress your workouts for continued improvement.
- Minimize injury risk through proper form and control.
- Maximize the effectiveness of your resistance band training.

Moving Forward:

This chapter provided a foundational understanding of resistance band techniques. Remember, practice makes perfect! Experiment with different techniques, incorporate them into your bodyweight exercises, and don't hesitate to seek guidance from a trainer or physical therapist for personalized recommendations. With dedication and this knowledge, you'll transform your workouts and unlock the full potential of your resistance bands!

Part 2

Targeted Workouts

Chapter 4

Upper Body Power: Arms, Shoulders, & Back - Build Strength and Confidence

Welcome to your upper body adventure! This chapter takes you on a journey to strengthen and sculpt your arms, shoulders, and back using the diverse power of resistance bands. Imagine toned arms, a strong core, and improved posture – achievable with dedication and the right exercises.

Targeting Key Muscles:

- **Biceps:** For those coveted "guns," bicep curls are your friend. Variations include standing, seated, hammer curls, and concentration curls.

- **Triceps:** The pushers of the upper arm, engage them with overhead presses, tricep extensions, and skull crushers.
- **Shoulders:** Sculpt defined shoulders with lateral raises, front raises, and reverse flyes, experimenting with different band positions.
- **Back:** Build a strong, supportive back with rows, pull-aparts, and seated cable rows, utilizing various anchoring points.

Sample Workout:

(Perform each exercise 10-12 repetitions, 2-3 sets, resting 30-60 seconds between sets.)

1. **Standing Bicep Curls:** Anchor the band under your feet, hold ends with palms facing up, and perform bicep curls.

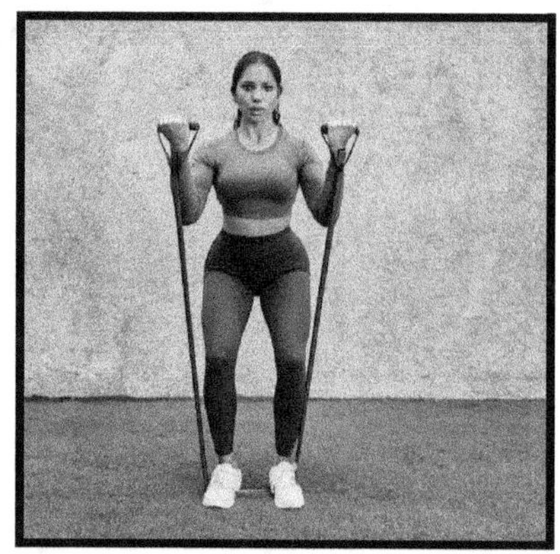

2. **Overhead Press:** Loop the band overhead, press your arms up, focusing on shoulders and triceps.
3. **Seated Rows:** Sit with the band anchored behind you, pull towards your chest, engaging your back muscles.

4. **Lateral Raises:** Loop the band around your ankles, stand with feet shoulder-width apart, and lift your arms out to the sides at shoulder height.

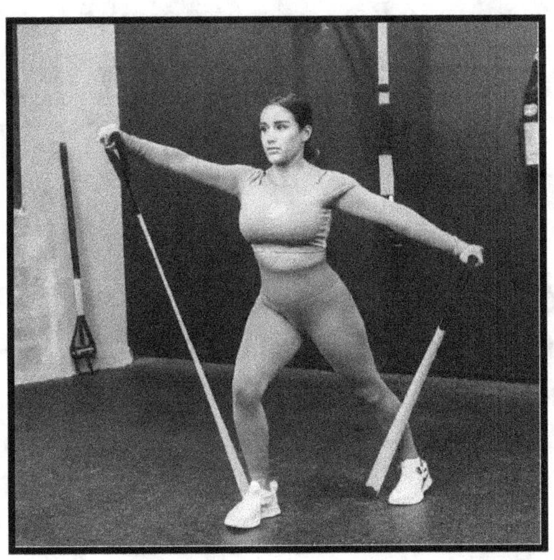

5. **Tricep Extensions:** Loop the band behind your head, bend your elbows with hands behind your head, and straighten your arms, engaging your triceps.

Remember:

- **Safety First:** Maintain proper form, listen to your body, and stop if you feel pain.

- **Warm-Up & Cool-Down:** Don't neglect these crucial steps to prevent injury and improve results.
- **Focus on Technique:** Feeling the targeted muscles is key to maximizing benefits.
- **Modifications:** Adapt exercises to your fitness level and limitations. Consult a professional for guidance.
- **Progression:** Gradually increase difficulty by using heavier bands, more repetitions, or adding variations.

Unlocking Your Potential:

- Explore advanced exercises like bicep curls with overhead press combo, band push-ups, and seated cable rows with rotation.
- Utilize different band anchoring points and grips to target specific muscle groups more effectively.
- Track your progress by recording sets, repetitions, and weights used to stay motivated and measure improvement.

Beyond Strength:

- Improved posture and balance.
- Increased bone density and reduced osteoporosis risk.
- Enhanced daily activities like carrying groceries or climbing stairs.
- Boosted confidence and self-esteem.

Embrace the Journey:

This chapter offers a roadmap to sculpting your upper body. Remember, consistency is key. Dedicate time to these exercises, experiment with different techniques, and celebrate your progress. With dedication and the empowering world of resistance bands, you'll unlock your full potential and achieve your fitness goals!

Remember, you are on a journey of self-discovery and empowerment. Enjoy the process, embrace the challenges, and witness the strength you build, both inside and out!

Chapter 5

Core Strength & Stability: The Powerhouse Within

Welcome to the core of your fitness journey! This chapter delves into the fascinating world of core strength and stability, the foundation for every movement we make. Think of your core as a powerhouse – a strong core supports your spine, improves posture, boosts balance, and enhances performance in all your activities.

Why Core Strength Matters:

- **Functional Movement:** A strong core allows for smooth, coordinated movements in daily activities and recreational pursuits.
- **Reduced Back Pain:** Core weakness often contributes to back pain. Strengthening your core improves stability and protects your spine.

- **Improved Balance & Stability:** A strong core enhances your balance, reducing the risk of falls and injuries.
- **Posture Powerhouse:** A strong core contributes to good posture, improving confidence and reducing strain on your back and neck.

Understanding Your Core:

Your core muscles encompass more than just your "six-pack." They include:

- **Transverse abdominis:** Deepest muscle, provides core stability and supports internal organs.
- **Rectus abdominis:** Familiar "six-pack," helps with trunk flexion and rotation.
- **Obliques:** Wrap around your sides, aid in trunk rotation and bending.
- **Erector spinae:** Run along your spine, support posture and movement.

Resistance Band Core Exercises:

This chapter introduces various exercises, with modifications for different fitness levels:

Plank Variations:

- **Basic Plank:** Forearms on the ground, body in a straight line, hold for 30-60 seconds.
- **Side Plank:** Lie on your side, elbow under shoulder, hips lifted, hold for 30-60 seconds each side.
- **Elevated Plank:** Use a chair or bench for your forearms for easier variations.

Crunches & Variations:

- **Standard Crunch:** Lie on your back, knees bent, lift upper back off the ground, engaging your core.
- **Bicycle Crunches:** Lie on your back, alternate bringing opposite knee and elbow towards each other.
- **Russian Twists:** Sit on the floor with knees bent, twist your torso from side to side, holding a band with both hands.

Anti-Rotation Exercises:

- **Plank with Arm Raise:** Hold a plank position, raise one arm at a time, maintaining core stability.
- **Dead Bug:** Lie on your back, arms and legs extended, slowly lower one arm and leg at a time, keeping your back flat.

Remember:

- **Focus on Form:** Proper technique is crucial to avoid injury and maximize effectiveness.
- **Engage Your Core:** Feel the muscles working with each exercise.
- **Start Slow & Progress:** Begin with easier variations and gradually increase difficulty as you strengthen.
- **Listen to Your Body:** Take breaks when needed and don't push through pain.

Beyond the Exercises:

- **Incorporate core exercises throughout your day:** Engage your core during everyday activities like standing and walking.

- **Maintain good posture:** Be mindful of your posture throughout the day to strengthen your core and improve alignment.
- **Consult a professional:** If you have any health concerns or need personalized guidance, seek help from a certified trainer or physical therapist.

Unlocking Your Potential:

- Explore advanced exercises like medicine ball slams, weighted planks, and band Palloff presses.
- Combine core exercises with other workout routines for well-rounded fitness.
- Track your progress and celebrate your achievements to stay motivated.

Building a Strong Foundation:

This chapter equips you with the knowledge and exercises to build a strong and stable core.

Remember, consistency is key. Dedicate time to these exercises, embrace proper form, and witness the incredible benefits a strong core offers. Embrace the journey, unlock your potential, and feel the power within!

Chapter 6

Lower Body Blast: Legs & Glutes - Sculpt and Strengthen Your Powerhouse

Get ready to blast your lower body and sculpt strong, toned legs and glutes with the magic of resistance bands! This chapter takes you on a journey to strengthen your foundation, improve balance, and boost your confidence, all while having fun with diverse and effective exercises.

Why Target Your Lower Body?

- **Functional Strength:** Strong legs and glutes power everyday activities like climbing stairs, carrying groceries, and maintaining good posture.
- **Improved Balance & Stability:** Strong lower body muscles contribute to better balance, reducing fall risk and enhancing agility.

- **Metabolic Boost:** Lower body exercises engage large muscle groups, burning more calories and boosting your metabolism.
- **Confidence & Power:** Toned legs and glutes can boost your confidence and self-esteem, making you feel strong and capable.

Understanding Your Lower Body:

Your lower body comprises various muscle groups:

- **Quadriceps:** Front of your thighs, responsible for extending your knees.
- **Hamstrings:** Back of your thighs, responsible for bending your knees.
- **Calves:** Lower legs, important for pushing off the ground and stability.
- **Glutes:** Large muscles on your buttocks, essential for power and hip movement.

Resistance Band Leg & Glute Exercises:

This chapter introduces a variety of exercises, with modifications for different fitness levels:

Squats: The king of lower body exercises!

- **Basic Squat:** Stand with feet hip-width apart, loop band around thighs, lower down as if sitting back, engaging glutes and quads.
- **Sumo Squat:** Wider stance, toes pointed outward, targets inner thighs.

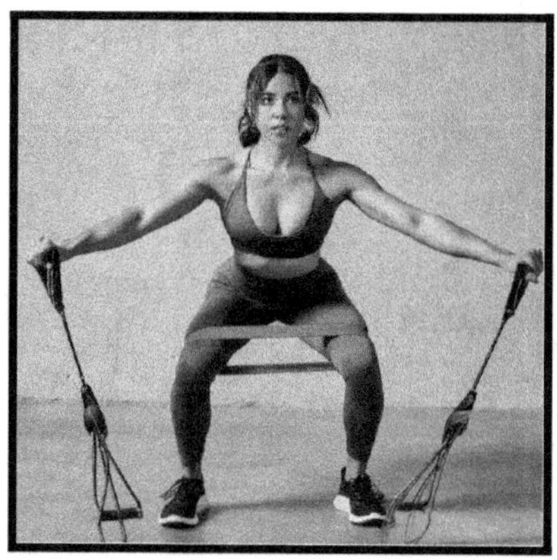

- **Chair Squat:** Use a chair for support, good for beginners.

Lunges: Work each leg individually and improve balance.

- **Forward Lunge:** Step forward with one leg, lower both knees, push back to starting position.
- **Reverse Lunge:** Step backward with one leg, lower both knees, push back to starting position.
- **Walking Lunges:** Continuous lunges, great for coordination.

Glute Bridges: Target your glutes specifically.

- **Basic Bridge:** Lie on your back, knees bent, feet flat, lift hips off the ground, squeeze glutes at the top.
- **Single-Leg Bridge:** Lift one leg while performing the bridge, challenging your balance.
- **Banded Bridge:** Loop band around thighs for added resistance.

Calf Raises: Strengthen and define your calves.

- **Standing Calf Raises:** Stand on toes, lower back down, engaging your calves.

- **Seated Calf Raises:** Sit on a chair, raise and lower your heels, focusing on calves.
- **Band-Assisted Calf Raises:** Loop band around the arch of your foot for added resistance.

Remember:

- **Warm-up and cool-down:** Prepare your muscles and prevent injury.
- **Focus on form:** Proper technique is key to maximizing results and avoiding injury.
- **Listen to your body:** Start slow, progress gradually, and don't push through pain.
- **Breathe throughout:** Maintain steady breathing during exercises.

Unlocking Your Potential:

- Explore advanced exercises like band walks, jump squats, and Bulgarian split squats.
- Combine lower body exercises with cardio routines for a complete workout.

- Track your progress and celebrate your achievements to stay motivated.

Beyond the Exercises:

- **Maintain good posture:** Stand tall and engage your core for optimal lower body alignment.
- **Stretch regularly:** Prevent tightness and improve flexibility.
- **Stay hydrated:** Drink plenty of water before, during, and after your workouts.
- **Consult a professional:** If you have any health concerns or need personalized guidance, seek help from a certified trainer or physical therapist.

Building Power and Confidence:

This chapter equips you with the knowledge and tools to sculpt strong, toned legs and glutes. Remember, consistency is key. Dedicate time to these exercises, embrace proper form, and witness the incredible benefits of a strong lower body. Feel the power surge through your legs, witness your confidence bloom, and enjoy the journey to a healthier, stronger you!

Chapter 7

Balance & Coordination Exercises: Mastering Movement with Confidence

Welcome to the realm of balance and coordination! This chapter unveils exercises with resistance bands to enhance your stability, agility, and overall movement confidence. Imagine navigating daily activities with grace and ease, tackling uneven terrain with poise, and feeling secure in your every step. With dedication and the right exercises, these goals become achievable!

Why Focus on Balance & Coordination?

- **Reduced Fall Risk:** Strong balance muscles and better coordination significantly reduce the risk of falls, especially for older adults.
- **Improved Daily Activities:** Enhanced stability and coordination lead to

smoother and safer movement in everyday life.

- **Enhanced Cognitive Function:** Studies suggest balance and coordination exercises can improve cognitive function and brain health.
- **Boosted Confidence:** Feeling stable and agile fosters confidence and independence, allowing you to enjoy activities fully.

Understanding Balance & Coordination:

Balance involves maintaining your center of gravity over your base of support, while coordination ensures smooth and efficient movement of various body parts. Both are crucial for safe and graceful movement.

Resistance Band Balance & Coordination Exercises:

This chapter introduces a variety of exercises, with modifications for different fitness levels:

Single-Leg Stances:

- **Basic Stand:** Stand on one leg for as long as comfortable, holding a band for support if needed.
- **Eyes Closed:** Progress to closing your eyes for an added challenge.
- **Reach & Sway:** Hold a band overhead and gently sway from side to side while standing on one leg.

Heel-Toe Walking:

- Walk forward, placing your heel directly in front of your toes with each step.
- Use a band held in front of you for balance if needed.
- Progress to walking backward or sideways for an extra challenge.

Side Shuffles:

- Loop a band around your ankles and shuffle sideways, maintaining good posture.
- Increase the distance between your feet for more difficulty.

- Add arm movements for an additional coordination challenge.

Band Walks:

- Loop a band around your ankles and walk forward, backward, or sideways, feeling the resistance engage your stabilizing muscles.
- Increase the band tension or walking speed for a greater challenge.
- Perform figure-eight patterns or walk over small obstacles for added complexity.

Remember:

- **Start slow and progress gradually:** Begin with easier exercises and build up the duration and difficulty as you improve.
- **Focus on safety:** Perform exercises in a safe environment and use a spotter or support if needed.
- **Listen to your body:** Take breaks when needed and don't push through pain.

- **Incorporate these exercises into your routine:** Regular practice is key to seeing results.

Unlocking Your Potential:

- Explore advanced exercises like balance boards, wobble cushions, and tai chi movements with resistance bands.
- Combine balance and coordination exercises with other workouts for a well-rounded fitness routine.
- Track your progress by noting how long you can hold stances or perform exercises, celebrating your improvements.

Beyond the Exercises:

- **Practice mindfulness:** Be present in your movements and focus on maintaining good posture and body awareness.
- **Engage in activities that challenge your balance:** Dancing, yoga, or even gardening can be beneficial.

- **Stay hydrated:** Dehydration can affect balance, so drink plenty of water throughout the day.
- **Consult a professional:** If you have any balance concerns or medical conditions, seek guidance from a certified trainer or physical therapist.

Building a Foundation for Stability:

This chapter equips you with the knowledge and tools to enhance your balance and coordination. Remember, consistency is key. Dedicate time to these exercises, prioritize safety, and witness the incredible benefits of improved stability and agility. Move with confidence, navigate your world with grace, and enjoy the newfound freedom these exercises offer!

Chapter 8

Flexibility & Stretching Routines: Unlocking Movement Freedom

Welcome to the realm of flexibility! This chapter unveils the importance of stretching and provides effective routines using resistance bands to enhance your range of motion, improve circulation, and prevent injuries. Imagine effortlessly reaching for high shelves, bending down with ease, and moving with grace and freedom – all possible through consistent stretching and the magic of resistance bands!

Why Focus on Flexibility?

- **Improved Range of Motion:** Enhanced flexibility allows for greater movement in your joints, making daily activities and exercise easier and more enjoyable.
- **Reduced Risk of Injury:** Tight muscles are more prone to strains and tears.

Stretching helps prevent these injuries and keeps you active.

- **Enhanced Posture & Alignment:** Improved flexibility contributes to better posture and alignment, reducing pain and discomfort.
- **Increased Blood Flow & Circulation:** Stretching improves blood flow to your muscles, delivering oxygen and nutrients, aiding in recovery and reducing stiffness.

Understanding Flexibility:

Flexibility refers to the range of motion in your joints and the extensibility of your muscles. Different factors like age, lifestyle, and activity level affect flexibility.

Resistance Band Stretching Techniques:

This chapter introduces various stretching routines with modifications for different fitness levels:

Static Stretches: Hold each stretch for 15-30 seconds, aiming for a gentle pull, not pain.

- **Hamstring Stretch:** Sit on the floor, loop band around one foot, gently lean forward, keeping your back straight.
- **Quad Stretch:** Stand on one leg, hold band behind your ankle, gently pull your heel towards your gluteus.
- **Chest Stretch:** Hold a band in front of you, palms facing each other, gently pull your arms apart.
- **Shoulder Stretches:** Loop band around your hands behind your back, raise your arms overhead, or perform arm circles with the band.

Dynamic Stretches: Move through controlled, fluid movements, gradually increasing range of motion.

- **Arm Circles:** Forward and backward arm circles with a light band, gradually increasing size and speed.
- **Leg Swings:** Swing each leg forward and backward, keeping your core engaged, using a band for support if needed.

- **Band Walks:** Loop a band around your ankles and walk forward and backward, activating leg muscles and improving range of motion.

Remember:

- **Warm-up before stretching:** Prepare your muscles with light cardio or dynamic stretches.
- **Breathe deeply:** Inhale and exhale slowly throughout each stretch.
- **Listen to your body:** Don't push through pain, and stop if you feel any discomfort.
- **Stretch regularly:** Aim for 2-3 stretching sessions per week for optimal results.

Unlocking Your Potential:

- Explore advanced stretches like yoga poses with band assistance, partner stretches, and self-myofascial release techniques.

- Combine stretching routines with your regular workouts for a holistic approach to fitness.
- Track your progress by measuring how far you can reach or bend comfortably, celebrating your improvements.

Beyond the Stretches:

- **Stay hydrated:** Drinking plenty of water keeps your muscles hydrated and flexible.
- **Maintain good posture:** Sitting and standing tall throughout the day can improve your overall flexibility.
- **Engage in activities that promote flexibility:** Activities like yoga, swimming, and dancing can be beneficial.
- **Consult a professional:** If you have any flexibility concerns or injuries, seek guidance from a certified trainer or physical therapist.

Building a Foundation for Movement Freedom:

This chapter equips you with the knowledge and tools to enhance your flexibility. Remember, consistency is key. Dedicate time to these stretches, prioritize proper form, and witness the incredible benefits of improved range of motion and graceful movement. Unlock your potential, embrace the freedom of movement, and enjoy the active lifestyle you deserve!

Remember, you are on a journey towards a healthier, more flexible you. Embrace the challenge, feel the tension release, and celebrate the newfound freedom in your movements!

Part 3

Taking it Further

Chapter 9

Advanced Workout Progressions & Modifications: Pushing Your Limits with Confidence

Welcome to the exciting realm of advanced progressions and modifications! This chapter equips you to elevate your resistance band workouts, challenge your muscles further, and personalize exercises to meet your unique needs and fitness goals. Remember, progression is key to staying motivated and seeing continuous improvement, while modifications ensure safety and cater to individual limitations. With this knowledge, you'll unlock a new level of fitness potential!

Why Progress & Modify?

- **Progression:** To avoid plateaus and keep challenging your muscles, gradually increase exercise difficulty. This leads to improved strength, endurance, and overall fitness.
- **Modification:** To ensure safety and cater to individual limitations, adapt exercises to accommodate injuries, fitness levels, or physical restrictions.

Progression Techniques:

- **Increase Band Resistance:** Use heavier bands or double them up for a greater challenge.
- **Increase Repetitions & Sets:** Gradually increase the number of repetitions and sets you perform for each exercise.
- **Shorten Rest Periods:** As your fitness improves, reduce rest periods between sets to keep your heart rate up and boost calorie burn.

- **Change Tempo:** Try performing exercises slower for more control and muscle engagement, or faster for increased agility and power.
- **Add Complexity:** Combine exercises, use unstable surfaces, or incorporate additional equipment for a more challenging workout.

Modification Techniques:

- **Reduce Band Resistance:** Use lighter bands or fewer loops to make exercises easier.
- **Decrease Repetitions & Sets:** Start with fewer repetitions and sets and gradually build up as your strength improves.
- **Lengthen Rest Periods:** Take longer breaks between sets if needed, listen to your body, and avoid overexertion.
- **Focus on Form:** Prioritize proper technique over heavier weights or faster speeds to prevent injury.
- **Choose Alternative Exercises:** Substitute exercises that are too challenging with

easier variations or ones targeting different muscle groups.

Remember:

- **Seek Professional Guidance:** Consult a certified trainer or physical therapist for personalized progression and modification advice.
- **Listen to Your Body:** Pay attention to pain signals and rest when needed. Don't push through discomfort.
- **Focus on Progress, Not Perfection:** Celebrate small improvements and be patient with your journey.
- **Warm-Up & Cool-Down:** Always warm up before and cool down after your workouts to prevent injury.

Sample Progressions:

- **Squats:** Progress from basic squats to single-leg squats, jump squats, or weighted squats with bands.

- **Lunges:** Start with walking lunges, then progress to stationary lunges, reverse lunges, or lunges with added weight.
- **Push-ups:** Modify by performing them on your knees, against a wall, or elevated on a bench. Progress to full push-ups, decline push-ups, or diamond push-ups.
- **Rows:** Begin with seated rows, then progress to standing rows, single-arm rows, or rows with added weight.

Sample Modifications:

- **Knee Pain:** Modify squats and lunges by sitting on a chair or performing wall squats.
- **Back Pain:** Choose exercises that don't strain your back, such as planks on forearms or seated rows with good posture.
- **Limited Mobility:** Adapt exercises to your range of motion, such as using smaller leg movements or modified arm positions.

- **Pregnant or Postpartum:** Choose low-impact exercises that are safe during pregnancy and postpartum recovery.

Beyond the Techniques:

- **Track Your Progress:** Monitor your workouts to see your improvements and stay motivated.
- **Find a Workout Buddy:** Having someone to exercise with can boost accountability and enjoyment.
- **Set Realistic Goals:** Set achievable goals that challenge you but don't discourage you.
- **Celebrate Your Achievements:** Acknowledge your progress, no matter how small, to stay motivated.

Unlocking Your Full Potential:

This chapter empowers you to personalize your workouts and push your limits safely. Remember, consistency and dedication are key. With the right progressions and modifications, you'll overcome challenges, achieve your fitness goals, and unlock a stronger, more confident you!

Remember, your fitness journey is unique. Embrace the challenge, personalize your workouts, and celebrate the incredible transformation you are achieving!

Chapter 10

Staying Motivated & Making Fitness a Habit: Fueling Your Journey to Success

Welcome to the crucial chapter on motivation and habit formation! This chapter equips you with the tools and strategies to stay fired up, overcome challenges, and seamlessly integrate fitness into your lifestyle. Remember, motivation ebbs and flows, but by building sustainable habits, you'll conquer plateaus and achieve long-term fitness success.

Why Stay Motivated?

- **Reach Your Goals:** Consistent effort is key to achieving weight loss, building strength, or boosting endurance.
- **Enjoy the Benefits:** Regular exercise improves mood, energy levels, sleep, and overall well-being.

- **Challenge Yourself:** Pushing your limits builds confidence and fosters a sense of accomplishment.
- **Live a Healthier Life:** Fitness reduces the risk of chronic diseases and promotes healthy aging.

Understanding Motivation:

Motivation is like a flame – it needs to be nurtured and rekindled regularly. Identifying your "why" and implementing practical strategies are key to staying lit.

Strategies for Staying Motivated:

- **Set SMART Goals:** Specific, Measurable, Achievable, Relevant, and Time-bound goals keep you focused and celebrate progress.
- **Find a Workout Buddy:** Partnering up adds accountability, support, and makes workouts more enjoyable.

- **Track Your Progress:** Seeing your hard work reflected in numbers or improved performance fuels motivation.
- **Reward Yourself:** Celebrate milestones with non-food rewards to reinforce positive habits.
- **Mix Up Your Routine:** Prevent boredom by trying new exercises, classes, or outdoor activities.
- **Listen to Upbeat Music:** Energetic music can boost your mood and energy levels during workouts.
- **Focus on Progress, Not Perfection:** Don't get discouraged by setbacks. Celebrate small wins and keep moving forward.

Making Fitness a Habit:

Habits are formed through repetition and positive reinforcement. Make fitness an automatic part of your day!

- **Schedule Workouts:** Treat workouts like important appointments and stick to your schedule.
- **Prepare Your Gear:** Lay out your workout clothes and equipment the night before to avoid excuses.
- **Find an Exercise You Enjoy:** Choose activities you genuinely like to increase the likelihood of sticking with them.
- **Start Small & Build Gradually:** Don't overwhelm yourself. Begin with manageable routines and gradually increase duration and intensity.
- **Make it Convenient:** Choose workouts that fit your lifestyle and schedule, like home workouts or gym routines near your work.
- **Join a Support Group:** Find a fitness community or online forum for encouragement and shared experiences.

Overcoming Challenges:

Life throws curveballs. Here's how to navigate them and stay on track:

- **Identify Your Triggers:** Recognize what derails your motivation and plan strategies to overcome them.
- **Don't Skip Workouts:** If you miss a session, get back on track the next day. Don't let one slip derail your progress.
- **Reframe Negative Thoughts:** Challenge negative self-talk with positive affirmations and reminders of your goals.
- **Seek Support:** Talk to your workout buddy, trainer, or therapist for encouragement and guidance.
- **Remember Your "Why":** Reconnect with your initial reasons for starting your fitness journey to reignite your passion.

Beyond Motivation:

- **Focus on the Long Game:** View fitness as a lifelong journey, not a quick fix.
- **Enjoy the Process:** Focus on the positive aspects of exercise, like feeling energized and empowered.

- **Celebrate Non-Scale Victories:** Track improvements in mood, energy levels, or strength, not just weight loss.
- **Make Fitness a Part of Your Life:** Find ways to integrate physical activity into your daily routine.

Unlocking Sustainable Success:

This chapter equips you with the knowledge and tools to stay motivated and make fitness a lasting habit. Remember, consistency and mindset are key. Implement these strategies, prioritize your well-being, and witness the incredible transformation in your life – both physically and mentally!

Sample Workout Plans for Different Fitness Levels with Resistance Bands

Important Note: These are just samples, and it's important to adjust them based on your individual fitness level, goals, and any limitations you may have. Always consult with a healthcare professional before starting any new exercise program.

Beginner:

Frequency: 2-3 times per week

Warm-up (5 minutes): Light cardio (jumping jacks, jumping rope), dynamic stretches (arm circles, leg swings)

Workout (30 minutes):

- **Squats:** 3 sets of 10-12 repetitions
- **Lunges:** 3 sets of 8-10 repetitions per leg

- **Push-ups (modified on knees if needed):** 3 sets of as many repetitions as possible
- **Rows:** 3 sets of 10-12 repetitions
- **Plank:** 3 sets of 30-60 seconds hold
- **Bicep curls:** 3 sets of 12-15 repetitions
- **Tricep extensions:** 3 sets of 12-15 repetitions

Cool-down (5 minutes): Static stretches (hamstring stretch, quad stretch, chest stretch, shoulder stretch)

Intermediate:

Frequency: 3-4 times per week

Warm-up (5 minutes): Same as beginner

Workout (45 minutes):

- **Squats:** 3 sets of 12-15 repetitions, add weight band for increased difficulty
- **Walking lunges:** 3 sets of 10-12 repetitions per leg
- **Push-ups (full push-ups if possible):** 3 sets of as many repetitions as possible

- **Overhead press:** 3 sets of 10-12 repetitions
- **Side plank:** 3 sets of 30-60 seconds hold per side
- **Single-leg Romanian deadlifts:** 3 sets of 8-10 repetitions per leg
- **Hammer curls:** 3 sets of 12-15 repetitions
- **Overhead tricep extensions:** 3 sets of 12-15 repetitions

Cool-down (5 minutes): Same as beginner

Advanced:

Frequency: 4-5 times per week

Warm-up (5 minutes): Same as beginner

Workout (60 minutes):

- **Jump squats:** 3 sets of 10-12 repetitions
- **Bulgarian split squats:** 3 sets of 8-10 repetitions per leg
- **Decline push-ups:** 3 sets of as many repetitions as possible

- **Arnold press:** 3 sets of 10-12 repetitions
- **Anti-rotation plank:** 3 sets of 30-60 seconds hold per side
- **Single-leg deadlifts:** 3 sets of 8-10 repetitions per leg
- **Concentration curls:** 3 sets of 12-15 repetitions
- **Close-grip bench press:** 3 sets of 10-12 repetitions

Cool-down (5 minutes): Same as beginner

Additional Tips:

- Choose a weight band that provides moderate to challenging resistance, where you can complete the desired number of repetitions with good form.
- Rest for 30-60 seconds between sets.
- Focus on proper form rather than speed.
- Modify exercises as needed based on your fitness level and limitations.
- Always listen to your body and take rest days when needed.

Remember, consistency is key. Stick with your workouts, gradually increase the difficulty as you get stronger, and enjoy the process of achieving your fitness goals!

Troubleshooting common aches and pains

It's great that you're thinking about how to prevent and address aches and pains while using resistance bands. Here are some tips for troubleshooting common issues:

General:

- **Warm-up and cool-down properly:** This prepares your muscles for exercise and helps prevent injuries.
- **Use proper form:** Incorrect technique can strain muscles and joints. Pay attention to your posture and alignment during each exercise.
- **Start light and gradually increase intensity:** Don't jump into challenging workouts too quickly. Gradually increase the resistance, repetitions, or sets to avoid overtraining.

- **Listen to your body:** Take rest days when needed and stop any exercise that causes pain.

Specific aches and pains:

- **Muscle soreness:** This is normal after a new workout. Apply ice for 20 minutes at a time, several times a day. Use over-the-counter pain relievers like ibuprofen if needed. Rest and stretching can also help.
- **Joint pain:** If you experience joint pain, stop the exercise and consult a doctor to rule out any underlying conditions. You may need to modify exercises or choose different movements that don't aggravate the joint.
- **Lower back pain:** Ensure you're engaging your core muscles during exercises, especially when lifting weights. Avoid exercises that strain your lower back, such as heavy deadlifts. If pain persists, consult a doctor or physical therapist.

- **Neck pain:** Maintain good posture during exercises and avoid holding your breath. If pain continues, consult a healthcare professional.
- **Headaches:** Stay hydrated and avoid dehydration headaches. If headaches persist, consult a doctor.

Additional tips:

- **Consult a certified personal trainer or physical therapist:** They can help you create a safe and effective workout program tailored to your needs and limitations.
- **Invest in comfortable and supportive shoes and clothing.**
- **Stretch regularly:** Stretching before and after workouts can help improve flexibility and reduce muscle soreness.
- **Stay hydrated:** Drink plenty of water throughout the day to stay hydrated and help your muscles recover.
- **Eat a healthy diet:** Eating nutritious foods provides your body with the

nutrients it needs to repair and rebuild muscle tissue.

- **Get enough sleep:** Adequate sleep is important for recovery and overall health.

Remember, it's always best to err on the side of caution and consult a healthcare professional if you have any concerns or experience persistent pain. By following these tips and listening to your body, you can help prevent aches and pains and enjoy your resistance band workouts safely and effectively.

Glossary

Sure, here is a glossary of terms commonly used in resistance band workouts:

- **Abdominal Press:** An exercise that strengthens the muscles in your abdomen, also known as crunches or sit-ups.
- **Bicep Curl:** An exercise that strengthens the muscles in the front of your upper arm, also known as a bicep raise.
- **Chest Press:** An exercise that strengthens the muscles in your chest, shoulders, and triceps.
- **Deadlift:** An exercise that strengthens the muscles in your lower back, legs, and core.
- **Glute Bridge:** An exercise that strengthens the muscles in your buttocks and hamstrings.
- **Hamstring Curl:** An exercise that strengthens the muscles in the back of your thigh.

- **Lateral Raise:** An exercise that strengthens the muscles in your shoulders.
- **Overhead Press:** An exercise that strengthens the muscles in your shoulders, triceps, and core.
- **Pull-Up:** An exercise that strengthens the muscles in your back, biceps, and forearms.
- **Push-Up:** An exercise that strengthens the muscles in your chest, shoulders, triceps, and core.
- **Row:** An exercise that strengthens the muscles in your back, biceps, and forearms.
- **Squat:** An exercise that strengthens the muscles in your legs, buttocks, and core.
- **Tricep Extension:** An exercise that strengthens the muscles in the back of your upper arm.

I hope this helps!

Bonus

Sample Workout Log Sheet

This is a simple and printable workout log sheet you can use to track your resistance band workouts. Customize it to fit your needs!

Date: ______

Workout: ______ (Name of your workout routine)

Warm-up (5 minutes):

- List the warm-up exercises you performed and any notes (e.g., sets, reps)

Workout (duration):

Cool-down (5 minutes):

- List the cool-down exercises you performed and any notes (e.g., sets, reps)

Additional Notes:

- Use this space to record any observations about your workout, how you felt, or any goals you set for next time.

Tips:

- Use different colored pens to track different muscle groups or workouts.
- Include rest times between sets.
- Track your progress by noting your weight, reps, and sets over time.
- Celebrate your achievements and milestones!

This is just a sample, feel free to adjust it to fit your specific needs and preferences. Don't forget to listen to your body and have fun!

Sample workout log sheet

https://docs.google.com/spreadsheets/d/15e_X4_SKcmbEKr88N-LhdVD5ma6yEe66-nPxdae9VEg/edit?usp=drivesdk

Link for sample workout log sheet

Bonus
Video link for tutorials